漫画中药故事系列

Chinese Medicines in Cartoon Series

君药传奇

（汉英对照）

Tales of Emperors and TCM
(Chinese-English)

杨柏灿　**主编**
Edited by Yang Baican

杨熠文　晋　永　鲍思思　祝建龙　◎**文/译**
Paperwork by Yang Yiwen, Jin Yong, Bao Sisi, Zhu Jianlong

孔珏莹　夏瑜桢　金潇逸　◎**绘**
Brushwork by Kong Jueying, Xia Yuzhen, Jin Xiaoyi

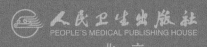

人民卫生出版社
PEOPLE'S MEDICAL PUBLISHING HOUSE

·北　京·

图书在版编目（CIP）数据

君药传奇：汉英对照 / 杨柏灿主编 . —北京：人民卫生出版社，2021.3

（漫画中药故事系列）

ISBN 978-7-117-31334-6

Ⅰ.①君… Ⅱ.①杨… Ⅲ.①中药材 – 普及读物 – 汉、英 Ⅳ.①R282-49

中国版本图书馆 CIP 数据核字（2021）第 038063 号

人卫智网	www.ipmph.com	医学教育、学术、考试、健康，
		购书智慧智能综合服务平台
人卫官网	www.pmph.com	人卫官方资讯发布平台

漫画中药故事系列——君药传奇（汉英对照）
Manhua Zhongyao Gushi Xilie——Junyao Chuanqi（Han-Ying Duizhao）

主　　编：杨柏灿
出版发行：人民卫生出版社（中继线 010-59780011）
地　　址：北京市朝阳区潘家园南里 19 号
邮　　编：100021
E - mail：pmph @ pmph.com
购书热线：010-59787592　010-59787584　010-65264830
印　　刷：北京顶佳世纪印刷有限公司
经　　销：新华书店
开　　本：889×1194　1/24　印张：3
字　　数：88 千字
版　　次：2021 年 3 月第 1 版
印　　次：2021 年 4 月第 1 次印刷
标准书号：ISBN 978-7-117-31334-6
定　　价：48.00 元

打击盗版举报电话：010-59787491　E-mail：WQ @ pmph.com
质量问题联系电话：010-59787234　E-mail：zhiliang @ pmph.com

序言

由上海中医药大学杨柏灿教授主编的《漫画中药故事系列》由人民卫生出版社出版了。这也是杨教授十年来从事中医药文化研究、作品创作和开展中医药文化普及工作的又一力作。

中医药是中国优秀传统文化的代表，凝聚着深邃的中国古代哲学智慧和科学文明的精髓。在抗击新冠肺炎疫情中，中医药发挥了突出的作用，引起世人的高度关注。国家的重视、社会的认同和关注，使中医药的发展迎来了前所未有的大好时机。抓住这一千载难逢的契机，做好中医药的传承与创新、推广与普及工作，是每一位中医药工作者义不容辞的责任。

做好中医药的传承、创新与弘扬，首先重在传承，只有真正做好传承，将中医药的精气神传承下来，才有可能不断创新、发展、弘扬。要做好中医药的传承，除了专业院校的教学以及师承以外，在全社会开展中医药知识的普及推广是一项十分重要的工作，特别是重视"从娃娃抓起"，从小就让我们的孩子沐浴中医药知识的阳光雨露，领略中医药世界的奥秘，感受中国传统文化的伟大，树立文化自信，使之入心入脑，有助于增强孩子们的民族自豪感，激发爱国情怀。

Foreword

Chinese Medicines in Cartoon Series compiled by Professor Yang Baican from Shanghai University of Traditional Chinese Medicine (SHTCM) is published by People's Medical Publishing House. It is a masterpiece by Professor Yang after his 10-year study on, writing about and popularization of Chinese medicine culture.

Traditional Chinese medicine (TCM) is representative of traditional Chinese culture, where lies the wisdom of ancient Chinese philosophy and the essence of scientific civilization. In the fight against COVID-19 epidemic, TCM has been playing an important role and attracts a lot of attention. Valued by the nation and accepted and followed with interest by the society, TCM has an unprecedented opportunity for development. It is a duty for every TCM worker to seize this opportunity and perform well in inheritance, innovation, promotion and popularization of TCM.

To inherit, innovate and carry forward TCM, inheritance is the first and foremost. TCM can be innovated, developed and carried forward only when it is inherited properly with its essence handed down. For inheritance of TCM, besides teachings in professional schools and from a master to his/her apprentices, it is important to popularize TCM knowledge in the whole society, with focus on "Starts with children". Let our children bathe in the sunshine of TCM knowledge, get to know the mystery of TCM and feel the magnificence of traditional Chinese culture, so that they can have cultural confidence, which helps enhance their sense of national pride and inspire their love for the country.

近年来，一些有识之士已开展了卓有成效的"中医药走进中小学"的工作，受到了广泛的关注和认同。伴随着国家综合实力的增强，我国国际社会地位的提升，中医药的国际影响力也日益扩大。重视中医药走向国际，弘扬中国传统文化，不但有利于提升我国文化软实力，而且也有益于中医药为全人类造福。

杨柏灿教授是上海中医药大学从事中药学教学的教师。他在完成中医药的医、教、研工作之余，十年来致力于中医药知识的推广与普及工作，在国内最早开设了中药慕课课程《走近中药》《杏林探宝——带你走进中药》《杏林探宝——认知中药》《中药学》《中药知多少》以及微视频《中药知识——走进中小学》。其中《杏林探宝——认知中药》上线美国 Coursera 平台，受众人群遍及 80 余个国家和地区，学习人数达 10 余万人次。同时，杨教授笔耕不辍，六年来先后出版了中医药通识读本《药缘文化——中药与文化的交融》《药名文化——中药与文化的交融》，连续三年出版了《本草光阴——中药养生文化日历》，在社会上产生一定的影响。

In recent years, men of sight have carried out projects of "Introducing TCM into middle and primary schools", which is widely concerned and approved. With enhancement of the overall national strength and the elevated status of China in the international community, TCM has an increasingly large international influence. Paying attention to international communication of TCM and carrying forward traditional Chinese culture can not only strengthen the cultural soft power of China, but also bring benefit for all mankind.

The author is a professor in Chinese medicines in SHTCM. After finishing his work as a doctor, teacher and researcher in TCM, he has been dedicated to promotion and popularization of TCM knowledge for nearly a decade. He is the first to provide MOOCs on Chinese medicines in China, including *Get Closer to Chinese Medicines*, *Hunt for Treasure in Apricot Grove — Bring You Closer to Chinese Medicines*, *Hunt for Treasure in Apricot Grove — Get to Know Chinese Medicines*, *Traditional Chinese Pharmacology* and *What Do You Know About Chinese Medicines*, as well as a micro video of *Knowledge about Chinese Medicines — Introduced into Middle and Primary Schools*. Among them, *Hunt for Treasure in Apricot Grove — Get to Know Chinese Medicines* is available online on Coursera, with audience from more than 80 countries and regions and learned by over 100,000 person-time. At the same time, Professor Yang has been writing continuously. In recent six years, he has published books on TCM including *Medicine Culture—Blending of Chinese Medicines and Culture* and *Medicine Name Culture—Blending of Chinese Medicines and Culture* and has published *Time and Chinese Materia Medica—Health Culture Calendar with Chinese Medicines*, which has a certain social impact.

《漫画中药故事系列》突破了目前市面上单纯以文字讲中药故事，或是将中药故事与中药知识相割离的作品形式，遍查古籍，选取有史实依据、民众知晓度高、具有深厚中国传统文化底蕴的中药故事，通过生动形象的漫画和精练朴实的语言，讲解中药故事，向世人展示中药知识与中国多元优秀传统文化的交融。读者在赏读本丛书时，不但能了解常用的中药知识，还能在不知不觉中接受中国传统文化的熏陶。本丛书的文字部分采用中英文对照的形式，益于中医药在国际上传播，同时也使中小学生在阅读漫画、接受中医药知识之余，提升英语的阅读能力。

本丛书的出版发行对于中医药的推广、普及势必有一定的促进作用，期待杨柏灿教授团队能不断有新的作品问世。

上海市卫生健康委员会副主任
上海市中医药管理局副局长
上海中医药学会会长
原上海中医药大学副校长

胡鸿毅

2020 年 9 月

Chinese Medicines in Cartoon Series gets rid of the layout of telling stories about Chinese medicines in words alone or separating the stories from the knowledge. The author has consulted ancient books and selected the stories that are based on historical facts, well known among people and deeply rooted in traditional Chinese culture. The stories about Chinese medicines are told through vivid cartoons and in simple language. They show the world the blending of knowledge about Chinese medicines with traditional Chinese culture, so that the reader can not only know about Chinese medicines, but also feel the charm of traditional Chinese culture. The text part of the series of books is in both Chinese and English to promote international spread of TCM, and additionally, the students in middle and primary schools can have their English reading ability improved while reading the cartoons and learning about Chinese medicines.

Publishing and distribution of this series of books will surely give an impetus to the promotion and popularization of TCM and I look forward to more works by the team led by Professor Yang Baican.

Deputy director, Shanghai Municipal Health Commission

Deputy director, Shanghai Municipal Administrator of Traditional Chinese Medicine

President, Shanghai Association of Traditional Chinese Medicine

Former vice-president, Shanghai University of Traditional Chinese Medicine

Hu Hongyi

Sep, 2020

心　人　牽　恙　微　有　帝
君　揚　藥　病　之　君　瘉
行　賤　貴　无　並　草　不
醫　藥　貴　須　非　病　君
臣　賜　酒　鴆　以　去
疢　療　可　亦　鵬　和　不

前言

Preface

随着我国综合实力的不断提高和国际地位的日益提升，文化软实力建设、树立文化自信，已成为国家的发展战略。习近平总书记指出"中医药学凝聚着深邃的哲学智慧和中华民族几千年的健康养生理念及其实践经验，是中国古代科学的瑰宝，也是打开中华文明宝库的钥匙"，高屋建瓴地概括了中医药在传统文化中具有不可替代的地位及其所具有的鲜明的文化特征。

《漫画中药故事系列》以历史悠久、扎根于中华大地、深植于大众心灵的中药为切入点，通过具有史料记载、民间知晓度高的典故传说，采用形象生动的漫画形式，传播中药知识，弘扬传统文化。丛书共分四册，既可独立成书又前后互为关联。

第一册《名医药传》：从中药雅称、药物应用、功效发现，介绍家喻户晓的名医名家治疗顽苛痼疾、疑难杂症的故事。

第二册《君药传奇》：从药名来历、药物应用等方面，介绍中药与古代君王间的趣闻典故以及民间医药高手不畏权贵、巧用中药的故事。

With its increasing comprehensive strength and growing status in the world, China's cultural soft power along with cultural confidence turns to renascent tendency. Chinese President Xi Jinping, once claimed that "Traditional Chinese medical theory is the gem of ancient Chinese science and philosophy, and also a key to the treasure of Chinese civilization", reconfirming the irreplaceable position and distinct feature of traditional Chinese medicine (TCM) in our culture.

Chinese Medicines in Cartoon Series aims at spreading knowledge of TCM and promoting our national culture. The series takes the well-known herbs as entry, tells fact-based tales and illustrates stories with pictures in comic format. The series includes four books, each being a sub-topic of TCM.

Book I *Tales of Doctors and TCM*: stories about miscellaneous and critical cases, mainly from the aspects of herbs' poetic names and efficacy.

Book II *Tales of Emperors and TCM*: stories about emperors and herbs, mainly from the aspects of herbs' naming and efficacy.

第三册《品读中药》：从汤羹、酒与豆腐发明的故事，介绍中药与饮食文化的渊源，体现药食同源的特性；通过益母草、王不留行、远志等中药名称来历的典故，体现中药药名的文化内涵。

第四册《智用中药》：从药物生长环境、采摘时节、药用部位、应用方式等对药效的影响，体现古今医药学家认识自然、应用自然的智慧。

随着国家对中医药工作日益重视以及在这次抗击新冠肺炎疫情中，中医药不可或缺的作用，重视做好中医药的传承、创新及推广已成为全社会的共识。特别是近年来，越来越多人意识到，要做好中医药的传承应该从小抓起，要重视中医药走进中小学的工作。正是在这样的大背景下，本团队经过 3 年多的努力，在人民卫生出版社的大力支持下，完成了以传播中药知识、弘扬传统文化为宗旨的漫画中药故事系列丛书。期望本丛书的出版发行，能有益于中医药知识和传统文化的传播。

Book III *Tales of Food and TCM*: stories about herbs and diet through the invention of soup, wine and tofu; stories about herbs and its name origin through the naming of motherwort, polygala, etc.

Book IV *Tales of Creative Use and TCM*: stories about herbs and efficacy, mainly from the aspects of herbs' living environment, growing seasons, plant parts and application.

With the increasing emphasis on the traditional Chinese medical theory and its indispensable role in the combat against COVID-19, the whole society has reached the consensus that the traditional Chinese medical theory should be inherited, innovated as well as promoted. In recent years, more and more people have realized that the inheritance of TCM should be cultivated since childhood and that TCM should be introduced into elementary education stage. Thanks to People's Medical Publishing House, our team, after more than three years' constant efforts, has completed this series of comic books on TCM. We are hoping that Chinese medicine and traditional Chinese culture can be promoted after its publication.

考虑到中西方文化背景的不同，在英语翻译上侧重于意译，而非直译，部分内容及标题中英文有所不同，须结合具体故事情节予以理解。

本丛书适用于广大中医药爱好者，特别是中小学生。同时，本丛书中英对照的形式也有助于在国际上传播、宣传中医药知识和中国传统文化，推动中医药国际化。

Owning to the cultural differences between the East and the West, some parts of the stories have been translated sense-for-sense instead word-for-word.

This series of books is written for Chinese medicine enthusiasts, especially primary and middle school students. Meanwhile, in the form of both Chinese and English, it helps to spread Chinese medicine knowledge and culture so as to promote its internationalization.

《漫画中药故事系列》丛书编委会

2020 年 7 月 25 日

Editorial Committee

July 25, 2020

目录
CATALOG

第一部分
治君之疾誉美名

治愈君王之疾绝对可以算上是大功一件，一些药物正是借治愈帝王之疾而名声大噪，为世人所知晓。

Part I
Gaining A Good Reputation by Treating the Emperors' Diseases

The cure of the emperor's disease could definitely be counted as a great achievement of the doctor. And with the wide spread news of the emperor's recovery, some of the drugs used in the therapy became well-known to the world.

君王赐名徐长卿
Cynanchum paniculatum and Li Shimin

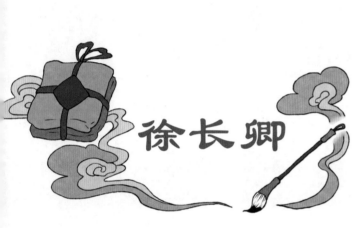

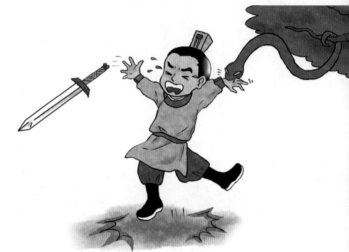

许多中药的命名与人名有关，中药徐长卿之名便是来源于一位古代医家，而这个名称更是由唐太宗李世民所赐。

Many names of traditional Chinese medicines are closely related to human's names. *Cynanchum paniculatum*, a certain kind of traditional Chinese medicine, is just one of the examples. It came from Xu Changqing, an ancient doctor, whose name was given by Li Shimin, Emperor Taizong of the Tang Dynasty.

相传在唐代贞观年间，太宗李世民外出打猎，不慎被毒蛇咬伤。

It is said that during the Zhenguan Period of the Tang Dynasty, Emperor Taizong Li Shimin was out hunting when he was accidentally bitten by a poisonous snake.

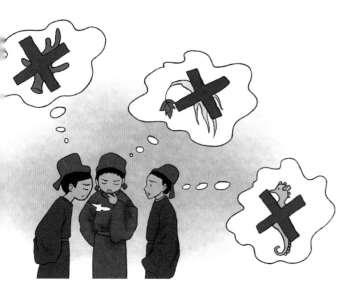

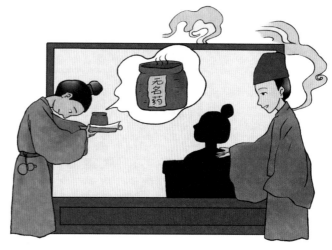

御医们穷尽许多贵重药材，但均不见效，只得张榜招贤。

Those imperial medics tried almost all the expensive and rare herbs, but still in vain, so they had to post a notice to recruit talents.

民间医生徐长卿看见榜文，便揭榜进宫为皇帝治病，他取三两自己采来的"蛇痫草"煎好，一日两次让李世民服下，余下的药液用作外洗。

Seeing the notice, Xu Changqing, a folk doctor, took it and went to the palace. He took out three liang (an ancient unit of weight) of "sheli grass" he had collected and decocted it. He ordered that most of the decoction be taken twice a day by the patient, and that the rest of it be used for external washing.

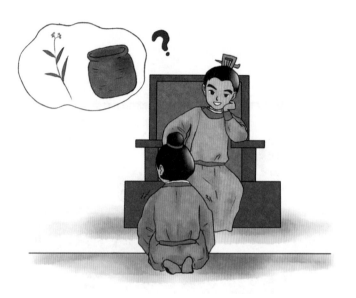

没过多久，中毒症状便完全好了，李世民喜出望外，便问此药之名，这时徐长卿却面露难色。

Before long, the poisoning symptoms completely disappeared. Overjoyed, Li Shimin asked Xu for the name of the medicine. Xu Changqing was a bit embarrassed.

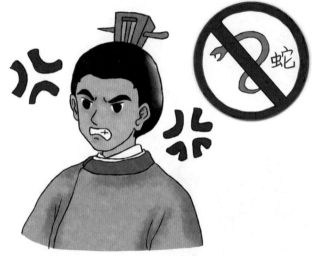

原来李世民被蛇咬伤后，下了一道圣旨，凡是带"蛇"字的都要忌讳，谁说了带"蛇"字的话都要治罪。

For after his accident, the emperor issued an imperial edict that anything with the word "she" ("snake" in Chinese) should be taboo and anyone who said anything with the word "she" should be punished.

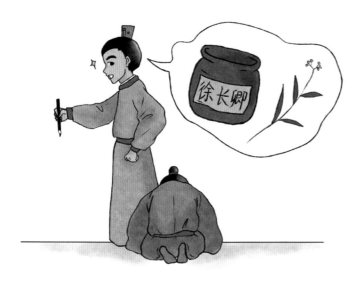

徐长卿便灵机一动说："禀万岁，这草药尚无名字，请皇上赐名。"皇上不假思索地说："是徐先生用这草药治好了朕的病，既不知名，那就叫'徐长卿'吧，以免后人忘记。"中药徐长卿的名字也就传开了，还一直沿用至今。

Suddenly, Xu Changqing had a brain wave. He answered, "Your Majesty, this herb has no name yet. Please give it a name." The emperor said without hesitation, "As Mr. Xu cured my illness with this unknown herbal medicine, let's call it 'Xuchangqing' in memory of you." The name of Xuchangqing, as a traditional Chinese medicine, spreads over till today.

徐长卿功效
The Efficacy of *Cynanchum paniculatum*

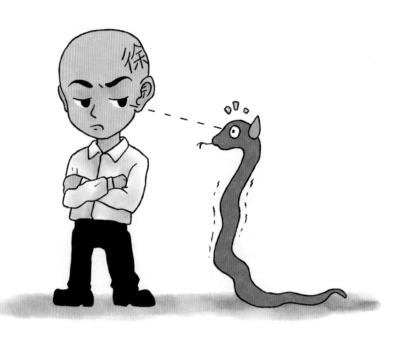

功效分析

蛇善行而灵动，其性与中医理论风邪的性质相似。徐长卿能够解蛇毒，根据取类比象推测其具有克制风邪的特性，其功效主要围绕祛风展开。风邪与湿邪常相伴为患，徐长卿可以祛风湿，治疗风湿痹痛；另外风胜则痒，徐长卿又可祛风止痒，用于荨麻疹等瘙痒性疾病的治疗。

Efficacy Analysis

Snakes are agile and good at crawling. Their nature is similar to that of wind-pathogen in TCM theory. Xuchangqing relieved snake venom, presumed that it had the characteristic of restraining wind-pathogen according to orientation analogy law. Its efficacy mainly centers on dispelling wind. Wind-pathogen and dampness-pathogen often accompany each other, and Xuchangqing treats rheumatic arthralgia by dispelling wind and dampness. In addition, as itches are often led by wind-prevailing, Xuchangqing is able to dispel wind and relieve itching to treat pruritus diseases such as urticaria.

君药同名刘寄奴

Artemisia anomala and Liu Yu

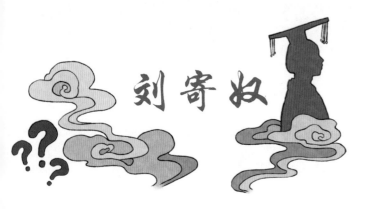

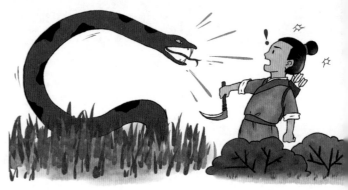

听到刘寄奴这个名字，或许你并不会联想到这其实是南朝宋开国皇帝刘裕的小名，不过可能令你更意想不到的是，它也是一味中药的药名，这究竟是怎么回事呢？

Hearing the name Liujinu (*Artemisia anomala*), you may not likely associate it with the nickname of Emperor Liu Yu, the founding emperor of the Song of the Southern Dynasty. What's more, what might surprise you most is that it also turns out to be a name of traditional Chinese medicine!

相传，一次刘裕在新洲砍伐荻草之茎时，一条长达数丈的大蛇突然窜了出来。

Liu Yu once was said to be cutting down the stem of the grass in Xin Land, when a huge serpent, as long as several zhangs (an ancient unit of length), jumped out.

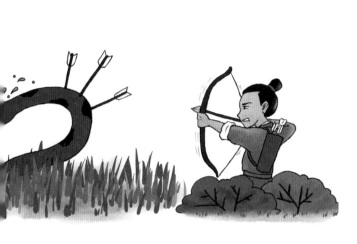

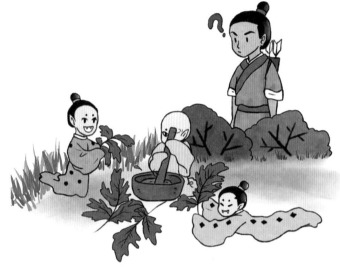

刘裕看见后并未惊慌，镇定地拉弓搭箭，射中大蛇，大蛇负伤逃走了。

第二日，刘裕又来到昨天遇蛇之地，发现有几个青衣童子在捣药，便上前询问。

Liu Yu, instead of panic, calmly drew his bow and shot the serpent. Wounded, the serpent narrowly escaped.

The next day, Liu Yu returned to the place where he met with the serpent, only to find several lads in cyan wrasse pounding the herbs.

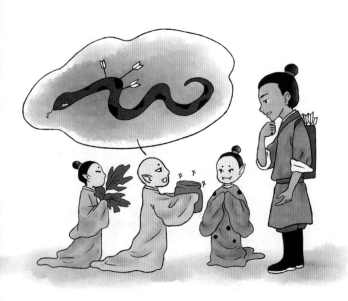

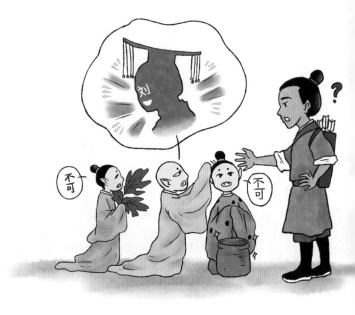

童子说："我们的大王被刘寄奴射伤，故遣我们来采药，敷于患处。"

The lads said, "Our master was shot by Liu Jinu, so we were sent to collect herbs and apply it to the wound."

刘裕奇怪地又问："那你们大王为何不吃掉刘寄奴呢？"童子回答："刘寄奴将来要做皇帝，乃不死之身，不能吃他。"

Liu Yu asked curiously, "Then why didn't your master eat him? " The lads replied, "Liu Jinu will be emperor in the future, so he should not die now."

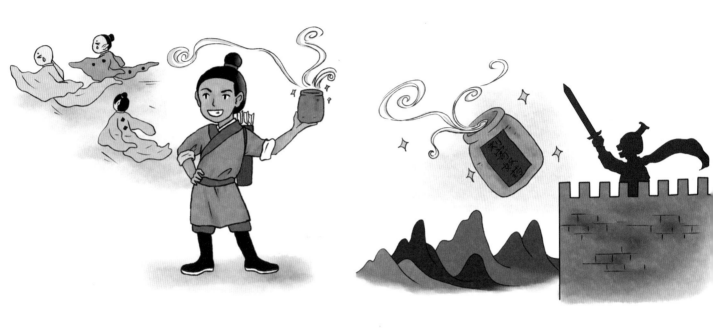

刘裕听后十分得意，便大声喝道："我就是刘寄奴。"童子们吓得弃药逃跑。刘裕便将那草药带了回去。

Liu Yu felt very proud after hearing the lads' words. He shouted, "I am the very Liu Jinu that you have talked about." Scared, the lads ran away, leaving all the herbs there. Therefore, Liu Yu picked the herbs up and took them back home.

后来，他果真成了宋武帝。每次领兵打仗，凡遇到将士被刀剑所伤，他便嘱其敷此药，甚是灵验，因而这药便得名刘寄奴。

Later, he did become Emperor Wudi of Southern Song Dynasty. Every time he led the troops to battles, he would treat his men injured by swords with the herbs. Just because of efficaciousness of this medicine, it got the name "Liujinu".

刘寄奴功效
The Efficacy of *Artemisia anomala*

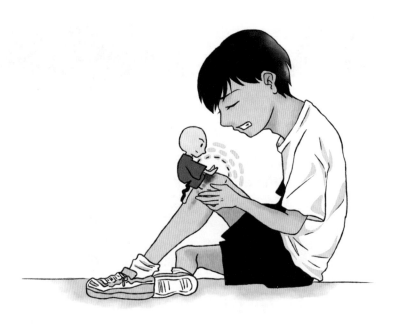

功效分析

从上文的传说中可知，刘寄奴具有疗伤的作用，能够用于跌打损伤的治疗。刘寄奴功用在于对血证的治疗，以活血为主，同时能够止血。故刘寄奴除了用于治疗刀剑创伤外，还能用于妇人经闭等其他瘀血病证。

Efficacy Analysis

According to the legend above, Liujinu has a healing effect and can be used to treat traumatic injury. Its main function is to treat blood syndrome, mainly by promoting blood circulation and stopping bleeding as well. Therefore, Liujinu can be used not only for treating stab wounds, but also for other blood stasis diseases such as women's amenorrhea.

以龙治龙道地龙
Earthworm and Zhao Kuangyin

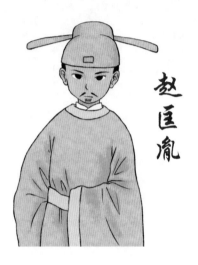

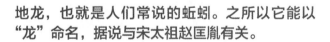

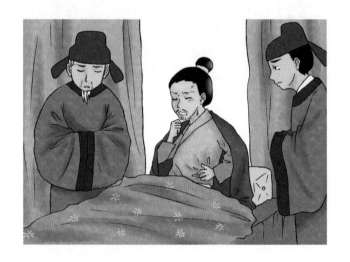

地龙，也就是人们常说的蚯蚓。之所以它能以"龙"命名，据说与宋太祖赵匡胤有关。

Ground dragon, also known as earthworm, got the name of dragon because it was believed to have some relation with Zhao Kuangyin, Emperor Taizu of the Song Dynasty (960-1279 AD).

相传在太祖登基后不久，他就患上了缠腰火丹，同时其哮喘病也复发了。

The legend goes that shortly after Emperor Taizu ascended the throne, he suffered from herpes zoster along with relapsed asthma.

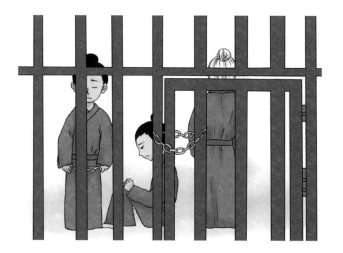

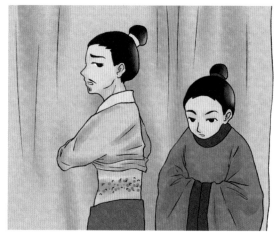

翰林院医官绞尽脑汁，也想不到回春之术。太祖一怒之下，就把所有医官监禁了起来。

The medics of the Hanlin Academy racked their brains, but still were not able to find the cure. Emperor Taizu was so furious that he imprisoned all the medics.

这时经医官推荐，一位民间郎中接旨前来宫中，他查看了太祖的病情，只见太祖环腰满是大豆形状的水疱，像一串串珍珠。

Just at that moment, upon the recommendation of a medic, a folk doctor came to the palace after receiving the imperial edict. When checking up the patient, he found around Emperor Taizu's waist some soybean-shaped blisters, like strings of pearls.

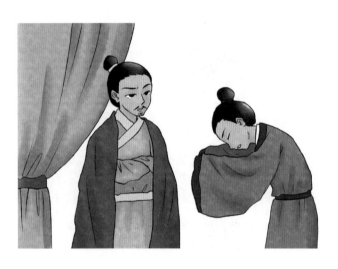

他和太祖说："这病不难治，如果治好了，希望皇上能够释放被监禁的医官。"太祖答应了他的要求。

He said to Emperor Taizu, "Your Majesty, your disease is curable. But would you please release all the imprisoned medics after your recovery?" Emperor Taizu agreed.

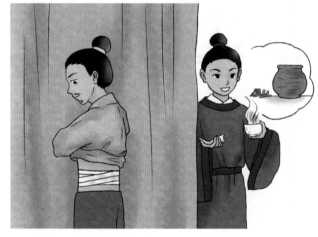

他从药罐中取出几条蚯蚓煎成药汤，一部分敷在患处，一部分则给太祖服下。

He then took out several earthworms from the medicine jar and decocted them in water. He applied some of the decoction to the affected part, and asked the emperor to drink up the rest of it.

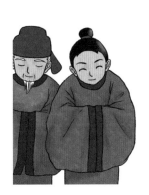
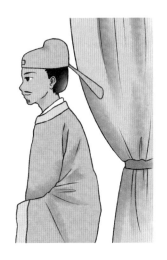
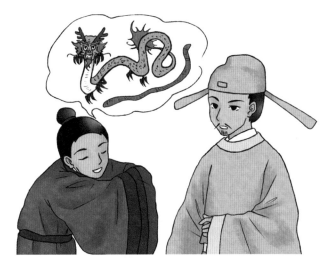

医治七天后，太祖的疱疹逐渐脱落，困扰多年的哮喘也痊愈了。

Seven days later, Taizu's herpes gradually fell off and the asthma that had troubled him for many years was also cured.

太祖好奇地问："这是什么药？"这位医家怕讲实话受到太祖责罚，便随机应变道："皇上是真龙下凡，这药叫地龙，以龙治龙，方能奏效。"

"What medicine is this?" Taizu asked curiously. Afraid of being punished by Taizu for telling the truth, the doctor answered indirectly, "Your Majesty, you are a real dragon and this medicine is called ground dragon. The medicine works when the two dragons meet."

地龙功效
The Efficacy of Earthworm

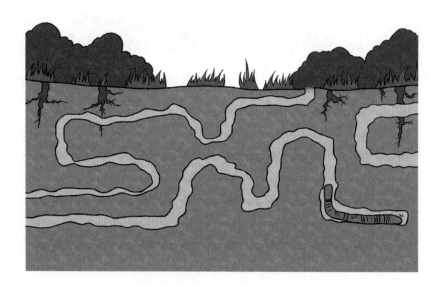

功效分析

地龙屈伸自如，穿行土中，故其性善通行，具有通行脉络，通利水道的功效，可用于脉络瘀阻、水肿、小便不利的治疗。同时，地龙又为血肉有情之品，长居于地下，秉阴寒之气，而可以清热息风止痉，用于高热不退、痉挛抽搐的病证。此外，如故事中所言，地龙兼具清热平喘的功效，外用还可治疗溃疡肿疮，只不过临床使用相对较少，也难怪文中医官将其淡忘了。

Efficacy Analysis

An earthworm flexes and stretches flexibly and travels through the soil, so its nature of being easy to pass through endows the effects of passing through veins and dredging waterways. It can be used for the treatment of vein stasis, edema and dysuria. Meanwhile, an earthworm is a creature of flesh and blood, living in the soil and holding the qi of yin and cold, so it can clear away heat to relieve wind and spasm, and thus it can be used to relieve the symptoms of high fever, spasm and convulsion. In addition, as mentioned before, an earthworm has both the effects of clearing heat and relieving asthma, and treats ulcer and sore through external application. However, these two clinical uses are relatively small, so no wonder that the medics had forgotten it in this story.

疗君扬名数阿胶
Donkey-hide Gelatin and Cixi

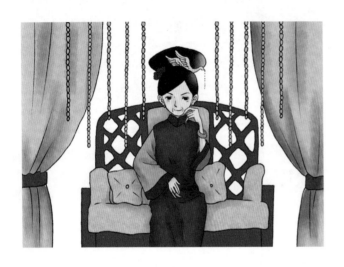

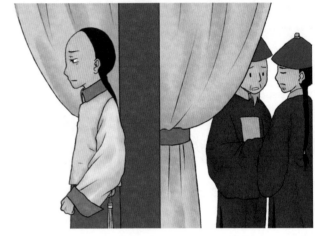

慈禧太后是清朝末年的实际统治者，她曾垂帘听政近五十载。而她与阿胶还有一段为世人称道的不解之缘。

Empress Dowager Cixi, the actual ruler in the late Qing Dynasty, who attended to state affairs for nearly 50 years, had an indissoluble bond with donkey-hide gelatin, an anecdote remembered by the generations.

清朝咸丰皇帝晚年无子，朝廷上下都很是焦虑。

Emperor Xianfeng of Qing Dynasty had no children in his later years, which worried the whole imperial court.

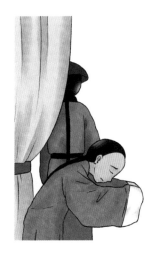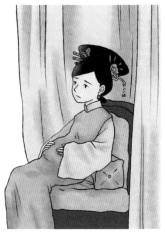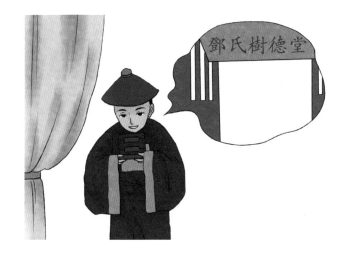

当时还是懿贵妃的慈禧好不容易怀孕，却得了"血证"，虽四处寻医，却都医治无效。

Empress Dowager Cixi, who was still Imperial Concubine Yi then, became pregnant at last. However, she got a "blood syndrome". Although she had received medical treatment in almost every way, she showed no sign of recovery.

这时，家居东阿的户部侍郎得知此事后，便献上城内"邓氏树德堂"所产阿胶。

The assistant minister of Revenue from Dong'e County got the news and offered Cixi donkey-hide gelatin produced by the local "Deng's Shude Pharmacy".

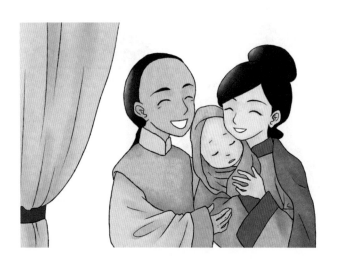

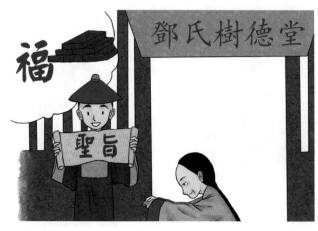

慈禧服用阿胶后，果真血证即愈，并足月产下一男孩，即后来的同治皇帝。

After Cixi took donkey-hide gelatin, she soon recovered from the blood syndrome and gave birth to a boy at full term, who was later Tongzhi Emperor.

得到慈禧产子的消息，咸丰皇帝大悦，赐予东阿阿胶"福"字，并封树德堂阿胶为"贡胶"。

Greatly delighted by the birth of the little prince, Emperor Xianfeng bestowed donkey-hide gelatin the word "fu" (good fortune) and conferred donkey-hide gelatin by Shude Pharmacy "imperial gelatin".

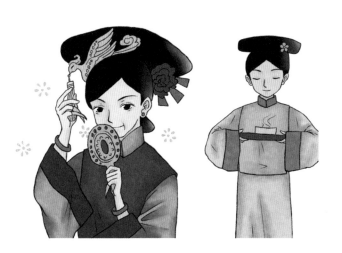

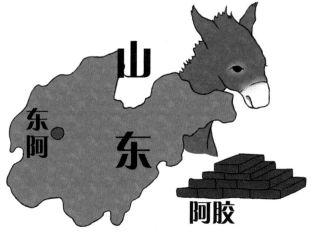

此后，慈禧常年服用阿胶，以至到了垂暮之年依然皮肤细腻润泽，不显老态。

Since then, Empress Dowager Cixi had been taking donkey-hide gelatin all her life, and even in her twilight years, her skin was still kept delicate and moist as young.

阿胶也借此声名远扬。阿胶由驴皮熬制成胶而成，因以出自山东东阿县为最佳，故名阿胶。

The donkey-hide gelatin became famous ever since. As it is made from the skin of a donkey, and the best products come from Dong'e County in Shandong Province, it has got the name Dong'e donkey-hide gelatin.

阿胶功效
The Efficacy of Donkey-hide Gelatin

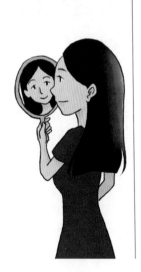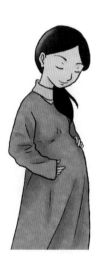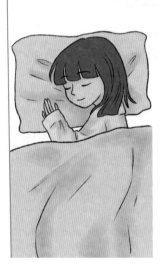

功效分析

慈禧所得的血证，相当于现代医学的"先兆流产"，以出血为主要表现，俗称"见红"，往往伴随有血虚。阿胶既能止血，又能补血，标本兼顾，是女性调经保胎的要药。同时，人的面色、毛发、肌肤也都赖于血液的滋润，血虚阴亏都会产生不同程度的问题，阿胶能够滋阴养血，自古以来便被视为养颜圣品。另外，对于肾阴不足，心血亏虚引起的失眠病证，阿胶亦具有补血安神，养阴除烦的功效。

Efficacy Analysis

The blood syndrome of Empress Dowager Cixi is equivalent to "threatened miscarriage" in modern medicine, with hemorrhage as the main manifestation, commonly known as "blood show" and is often accompanied by blood deficiency. Donkey-hide gelatin can stop bleeding, and enrich blood as well, taking into account of the root cause and symptoms of a disease. It is taken as an essential medicine for women to regulate menstruation, and protect fetus. At the same time, as people's complexion, hair and skin depend on the nourishing of blood, blood deficiency and yin deficiency will cause problems to varying degrees. Donkey-hide gelatin can nourish yin and blood, and has been regarded as a beauty-nourishing holy product since ancient times. In addition, donkey-hide gelatin also has the effects of enriching blood, tranquilizing mind, nourishing yin and relieving restlessness for insomnia caused by deficiency of kidney yin and heart blood.

第二部分
君病非须贵药医

在古代，虽然把君王身体视为龙体，但并非说必须以名贵药材才可医治，有时候一些平常普通的中药反而会取得更好的疗效。

Part II
Curing Emperors With Inexpensive Medicine

Although emperors are valued as dragons, it does not mean that they must be treated with precious medicines. Sometimes some common traditional Chinese medicines can achieve even better curative effects.

天麻止痛曹操鸡
Gastrodia elata and Cao Cao

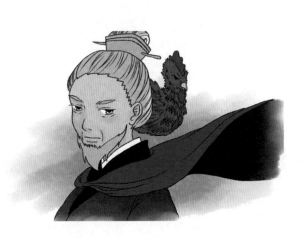

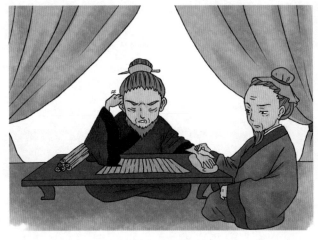

说到曹操，很自然会联想到他卓越的政治谋略，殊不知曹操还是一个美食家，对吃鸡尤有心得，并促成了一道药膳鸡的发明。

Speaking of Cao Cao, you will most probably think of his outstanding political strategy. However, few people would know that Cao Cao was also a gourmet with particular favor over chicken, contributing to an invention of an herbal chicken dish.

曹操常年患头风病，每因疲劳、紧张、愤怒便头痛加剧。

Cao Cao suffered from head wind disease all the year round. Every time he got tired, nervous and angry, his headache would become worse.

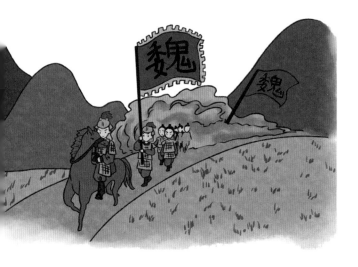

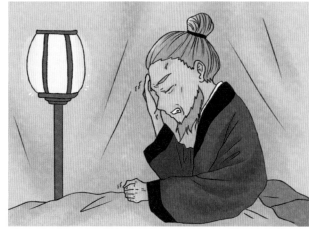

相传，建安十三年，曹操在统一北方后，率大军兴师南下伐吴。

In the 13th year of Jian'an, Cao Cao once led his army to attack Wu after preserving unity in the north.

行至庐州，因舟车劳顿，过度疲乏，曹操的头风病又犯了，寝食难安。

Arriving at Lu Land, Cao Cao again began to suffer from head wind disease due to excessive fatigue from the long journey. He was even unable to sleep.

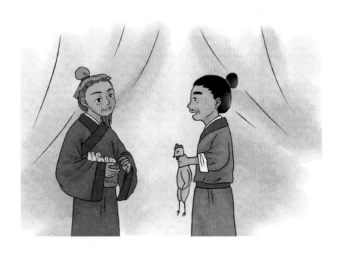

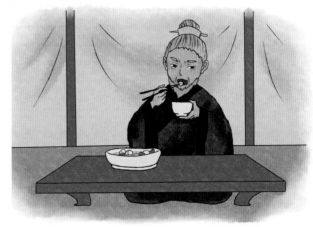

膳房的厨师素知曹操爱吃鸡，便以鸡为主料，并将随军医官的药方融入其中，共同烹制了一道药膳鸡。

The chefs in the kitchen knew that Cao Cao loved to eat chicken, so they took chicken as the main ingredient and mixed it with the medicines in the prescriptions by military medics, thus making an herbal chicken dish for him.

曹操品尝后感觉味道十分鲜美，待半只鸡下肚后，头痛也减轻了不少。

It was super delicious! After taking a half of the chicken, Cao Cao felt that his headache was relieved a lot!

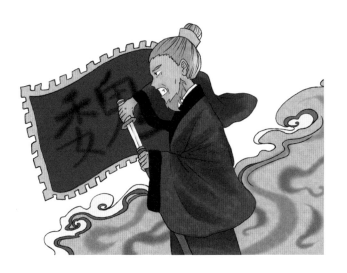

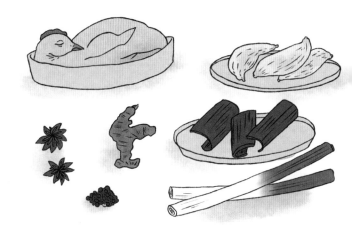

自此，曹操每次出征都会命膳房烹制这道鸡，这道药膳鸡也因此得名"曹操鸡"。

Since then, Cao Cao ordered his chefs to cook this herbal chicken dish every time he went out to battle, hence the name "Cao Cao chicken".

这道药膳鸡的关键就在于军医官处方中的一味中药——天麻。

The secret of this herb chicken dish lies in *Gastrodia elata*, a traditional Chinese medicine in the medic's prescription.

天麻功效
The Efficacy of *Gastrodia elata*

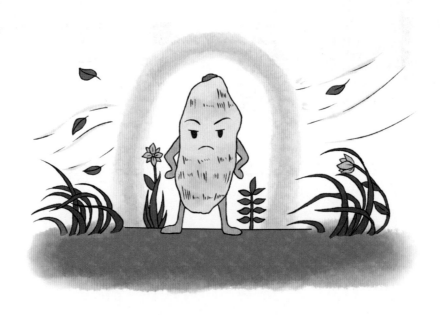

功效分析

头风病主要原因在于"风"对头部的侵袭，以致脑络不畅，不通则痛。因此，头风病的治疗须从祛风、通络、止痛三个环节入手。天麻被誉为"定风神草"，自然界中的天麻"有风不动，无风自摇"，其祛风之功可见一斑。且其性质平和，没有明显寒热偏性，作为药膳长期服用更是再合适不过。天麻还有显著的通络止痛功效。因此，是治疗如曹操"头风痛"的要药。目前认为天麻具有平肝息风、通络止痛的功效，主要用于头痛、眩晕等病证的治疗。

Efficacy Analysis

The main cause of head wind disease is the invasion of the "wind" on the head, resulting in poor cerebral collaterals and pain if blockage occurs. Therefore, the treatment of head wind disease must start from three aspects: dispelling wind, dredging collaterals and relieving pain. *Gastrodia elata* is known as the "wind-fixing magical grass". In nature, *Gastrodia elata* does not move in the wind, but shakes itself when there is no wind, so its function of dispelling wind is evident. Moreover, it is mild in nature and has no obvious cold-heat bias, so it can be taken for a long time as a medicated diet. *Gastrodia elata* also has remarkable effects of dredging collaterals and relieving pain. Therefore, it is an essential medicine for the treatment of "headache pain", as seen in Cao Cao's case. At present, *Gastrodia elata* is believed to have the effects of calming liver wind, dredging collaterals and relieving pain, and is mainly used for treating headache, vertigo and other diseases.

山楂消食糖葫芦

Hawthorn and Emperor Guangzong of the Song Dynasty

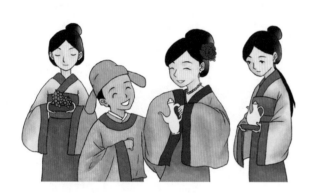

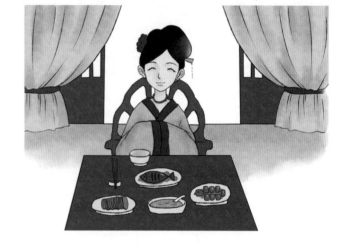

宋光宗是历史中典型的昏君，不思朝政、沉迷酒色，宋朝自他起也走向了下坡路。不过他与爱妃的小插曲却促成了糖葫芦的发明。

Emperor Guangzong of the Song Dynasty, a typical fatuous emperor in history, did not think of state affairs and became addicted to debauchery, directly resulting in the decay of the country. However, an incident between him and his concubine led to the invention of sugar gourd.

相传南宋时期，在一次宴会后，宋光宗爱妃突然得了怪病。

Once in the Southern Song Dynasty, one of Emperor Guangzong's beloved concubines suddenly fell ill after a banquet.

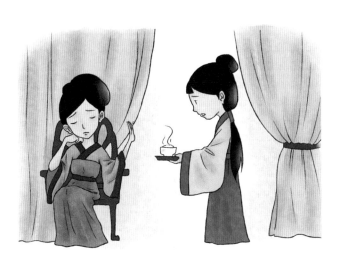

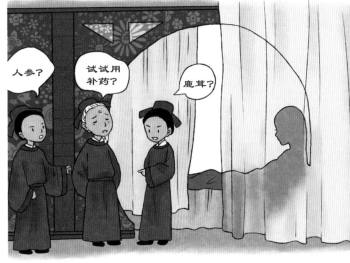

爱妃感到腹部胀痛，茶饭不思，身体也日渐消瘦起来。

She felt pain in the abdomen, had no appetite, and accordingly became weak day after day.

在朝御医皆认为这是体虚所致，用了大量补品，但都未见好转，光宗眼见爱妃身体一天不如一天……

The imperial medics in the court all believed that this was due to physical weakness, so they used a lot of supplements. However, none of them worked. Emperor Guangzong could do nothing but witness his beloved one getting worse and worse each day.

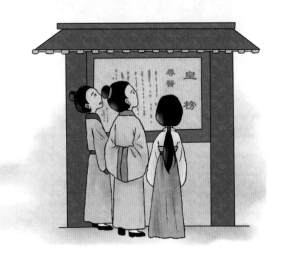

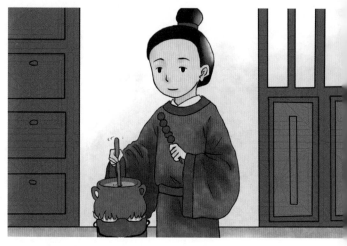

宋光宗十分焦急，无奈之下只得张榜寻医，此时有位江湖郎中揭榜进宫。

In despair, Emperor Guangzong had to put up a notice for talents. A folk doctor saw the notice and entered the palace.

在为贵妃诊脉后，他却说："贵妃的病并不重，只需用山楂与冰糖一起熬制，每顿吃五六枚即可。"听完后，宋光宗有些恼火，当朝太医用了这么多名贵药材都没用，这普普通通的山楂又能如何。

After feeling the pulse for the concubine, he said, "The disease is not so serious. What we need to do is just to boil some hawthorn with crystal sugar and serve the patient with five or six pieces for each meal." After hearing this, Emperor Guangzong was a little annoyed. "How can the ordinary hawthorn, far less expensive than so many valuable medicines the imperial medics prescribed, be effective?" he doubted.

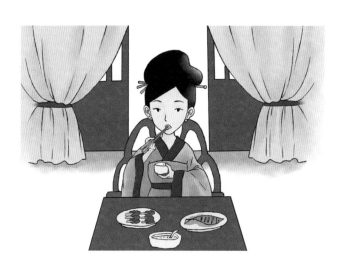

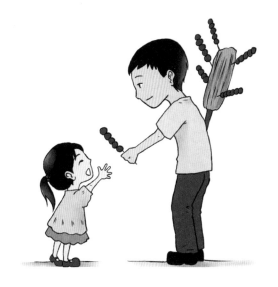

但苦于没有办法，便按照郎中的要求给贵妃服下。果不其然，爱妃吃后，胃口逐渐开始好了起来，不多久便恢复了往日的美貌。

As it seemed to be the only choice, Emperor Guangzong had to follow the doctor's advice. After taking the hawthorn several times, the concubine began to regain her appetite and gradually her former beauty as well.

后来，山楂这种做法流传到了民间，老百姓把它一个一个串起来，形成如今的街边美食——糖葫芦。

Later, the hawthorn recipe widely spread to civil society. People strung it up one by one, forming today's street food—sugar gourd.

山楂功效
The Efficacy of Hawthorn

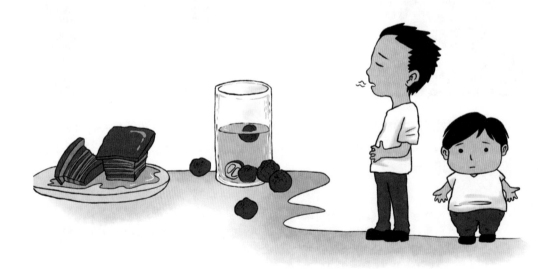

功效分析

从贵妃的病证来看，并没有明显的发展过程，主要与参与的宴会有关。因而，贵妃得病是由于过食而损伤脾胃，治疗应当从消化积滞的饮食入手，单纯补益反而会增加脾胃负担。山楂一药长于消食化积，作用强而应用广，无论是过食高脂肪、高蛋白的肉积，还是过食米面的谷积、面积都可以应用。同时，山楂甘酸开胃，亦可起到健脾养胃的功效。此外，山楂还具有活血化瘀的功效，现代还用于一些如高脂血症、肥胖等代谢性疾病的治疗。

Efficacy Analysis

Judging from the disease and syndrome of imperial concubine, we can see that there was no obvious development process. The disease was most likely related to the banquet. Therefore, her illness might have been caused by overeating, which later did harm to the spleen and stomach. The treatment should start with relieving dyspepsia, as simple invigoration will increase the burden on the spleen and stomach. Hawthorn is good at relieving dyspepsia with strong effect and wide application. It can be applied to meat-type food accumulation by eating high fat and protein food or grain-type food accumulation of over eating cereal and rice. In addition, hawthorn is sweet and sour for appetizing. It can also nourish the spleen and stomach. Besides, hawthorn has the effect of promoting blood circulation and removing blood stasis, so it is also used for treating metabolic diseases such as hyperlipidemia, obesity and the like in modern times.

丁香驱味口香糖
Clove and Wu Zetian

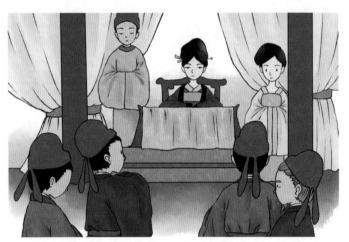
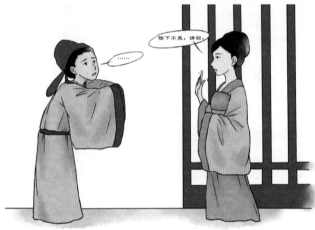

有口气是件令人尴尬的事，既苦于其味，又不便明说。中国历史上唯一正统的女皇帝——武则天便因此与中药丁香有过一段趣闻轶事。

Bad breath is embarrassing, and patients who suffer from it always feel ashamed to mention it. However, thanks to bad breadth, Wu Zetian, the only female emperor in Chinese history, had an interesting anecdote with clove.

相传，唐代宫廷诗人宋之问，仪表堂堂又满腹经纶，理应受到武则天青睐，可事与愿违，武则天却总是对他不理不睬，避而远之。

Song Zhiwen, a court poet of the Tang Dynasty, was handsome and knowledgeable, who as expected should deserve Wu Zetian's favor. But unfortunately, he was always ignored by Wu. And the latter even avoided seeing him several times.

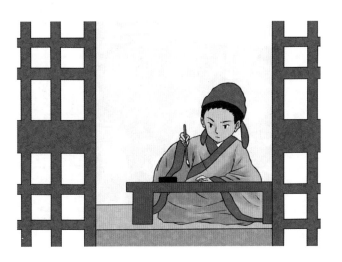

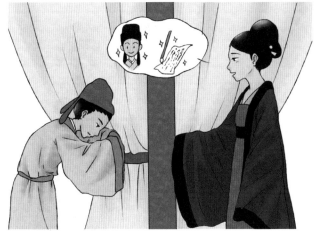

宋之问百思不解，于是便写诗呈现给武则天以期能够得到重视。

Song Zhiwen was very much puzzled, so he wrote poems to Wu Zetian in the hope to get attention.

武则天看了后，对他说："宋爱卿的诗文仪表都很不错，只是……"

After reading, Wu Zetian said to him, "My dear Song, you are a good-looking man with talents, but ..."

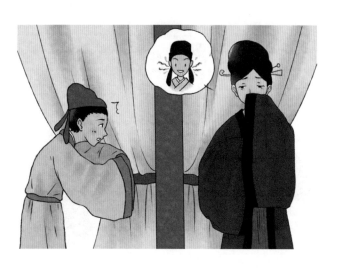

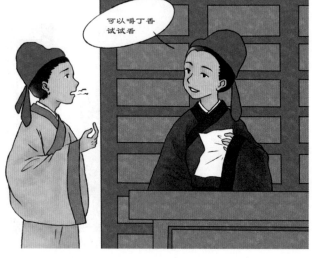

"只是爱卿不知道你有口臭这个毛病。"武则天捂着鼻子补充说。

"But don't you know that you have bad breath?" Wu Zetian added, covering her nose.

宋之问听后羞愧无比，就向太医询问解决办法，太医说："你可以嚼一嚼丁香试试看。"

On hearing that, Song Zhiwen felt extremely ashamed. He then turned to the imperial medic for help, who suggested he try chewing cloves.

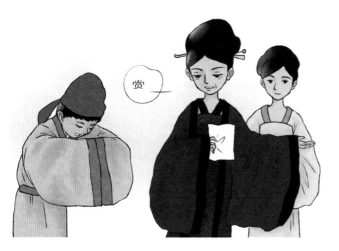

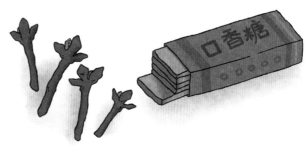

此后，宋之问每次出门时，嘴里始终含着丁香，渐渐武则天对他的态度也改变了许多。

Since then, Song Zhiwen always had cloves in his mouth every time he went out, and he gradually regained Wu Zetian's favor.

由此，有人也趣称丁香为世界最早的"口香糖"。

Hence, the clove is playfully referred to as the world's first "chewing gum".

丁香功效
The Efficacy of Clove

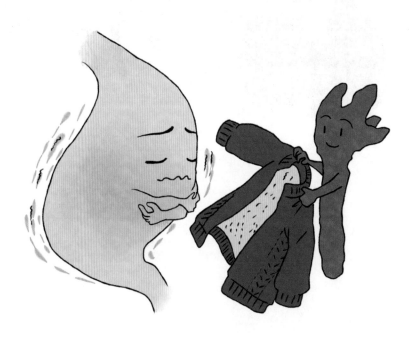

功效分析

丁香为日常所用的香料之一，其性芳香，故嚼丁香可以起到去除口气的作用。丁香作为药用，属于温里药，能够温中降逆、散寒止痛，用于胃寒呕吐、脘腹冷痛等病证；又可温肾助阳，用于男子肾虚阳痿、女子宫寒不孕的治疗。不过需要指出的是，中医一般认为，口气多由胃火引起，因此丁香除口气只能口嚼，不能吞服，不然反而会火上浇油，加重口气。

Efficacy Analysis

Clove, whose fragrance can cover up the bad smell, is one of the common spices used in daily life. Clove belongs to the medicine for warming the interior. It can warm the middle energizer and lower the adverse flow of qi, dispel cold and relieve pain, and is mainly used for treating stomach cold vomiting, abdominal cold pain and other diseases. It can also warm the kidney and activate yang to treat impotence due to kidney deficiency in men and infertility due to cold in women's uterus. However, it should be pointed out that traditional Chinese medical theory generally believes that the bad breath is mostly caused by the stomach fire, so clove can only be chewed but not be swallowed, otherwise it will add fuel to the fire and aggravate the bad breath.

第三部分
毒药致命亦疗疾

古代君王常以毒酒赐死身边的近臣、妃子。不过所用的毒物，其实亦属治病救人的中药之列。可谓是"用之不当，损人寿命；用之得当，可起沉疴"。

Part III
Healing Efficacy of Poisonous Herbs

In ancient times, emperors often killed their courtiers and concubines with poisoned wine. However, the poisons are also the traditional Chinese medicines taken to cure diseases and save lives. It proves the fact that improper use of TCM shortens life, while proper, sees full recovery.

李煜致死因马钱

Strychnos and Li Yu

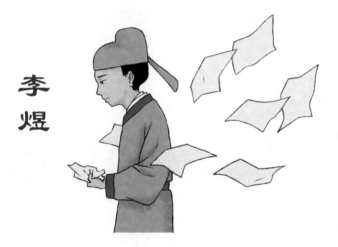

李煜

李煜是南唐最后一位皇帝，世称"李后主"。在历代帝王中，他是最有才华者之一，结局却最为悲惨。

Li Yu, the last emperor of the Southern Tang Dynasty, was known as "Li Houzhu". He is one of the most talented emperors in all dynasties, who yet ended his life in a most miserable way.

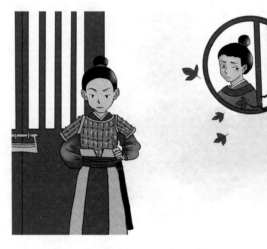

公元 975 年，宋军攻克金陵城，南后主李煜被俘，囚禁于宫中。

In 975 AD, Song troops occupied Jinling, the capital of the Southern Tang Dynasty, and Li Yu, the last emperor, was captured and imprisoned in the palace.

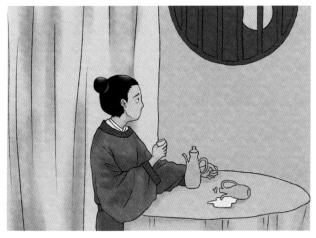

春花秋月何時了

往事知多少

小樓昨夜又[東]風

故國[不堪回]首[月明中]

雕欄[玉砌]應猶在

只是朱顏改

問君能有幾多愁

恰似一江春水向東流

囚禁期间，李煜日日借酒消愁。中秋之夜，李煜对酒赏月，不禁触景生情，勾起了对往事的怀念。

During his imprisonment, Li Yu drowned his sorrows to wine every day. On the night of the Mid-Autumn Festival, drinking in the moonlight, Li Yu got heartbroken, for everything he saw brought him back into memories of the past.

于是他提笔写下了千古传诵的《虞美人》："春花秋月何时了，往事知多少……"

So he wrote down the *Beauty Yu* which has been read through all ages: "When will the endless cycle of the spring flower and the autumn moon come to an end? How much remembrance of the things past does a heart know ... "

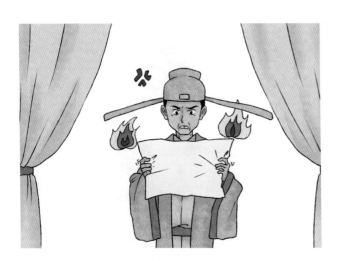

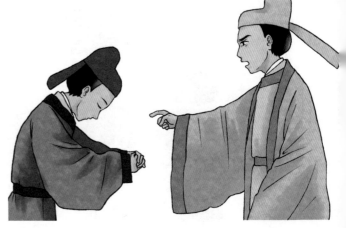

这首词传到了宋太宗手中，令其大为恼火，认为李煜并未丧志，还有着复国之心。

This poem definitely infuriated Emperor Taizong, who judged from the lines that Li Yu still had his ambition to restore his country.

于是宋太宗便借机赐以"牵机酒"，意图将其毒死。

So Emperor Taizong of Song sent him a jug of "Qianji wine" (main ingredients is strychnos), intending to poison him.

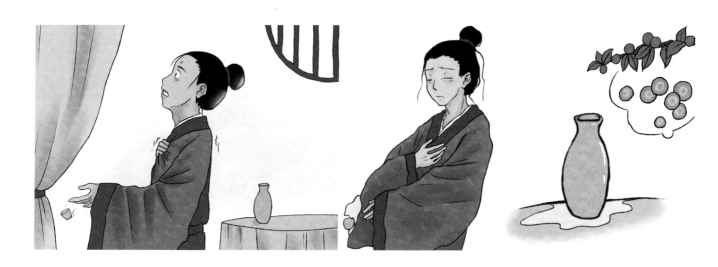

李煜并未察觉，酒至半酣，忽然全身抽搐，呼吸困难，不久便魂归西去。

Unaware of Emperor Taizong's maliciousness, Li Yu took the wine. He was about to be half drunk when his whole body suddenly began to twitch. With great breath difficulty, Li died very soon.

在这牵机酒中所用之药便是马钱子。

The medicine used in this Qianji wine is strychnos.

马钱子功效
The Efficacy of Strychnos

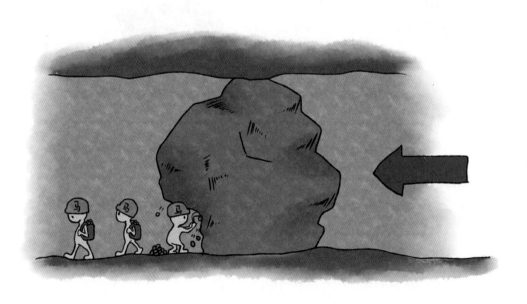

功效分析

马钱子以毒闻名，也以毒为用。从其"牵机药"之别名来看，服之死状如牵机，是一种肢体过屈反张的表现。因此可联想到，小剂量的马钱子可以起到通络的作用。而其应用也主要围绕通行二字，对于络脉不通的病证，马钱子能够开通经络，畅通气血；对于毒素堆积引起的癌毒痈疽，马钱子亦可通行散结消肿。

Efficacy Analysis

Strychnos is famous for its toxicity and is therefore used for toxicity. It is also known as "Qianji Drug". As the name of "Qianji" tells, the victim seems to be a stooped man, which is a manifestation of stretching instead of bending too much. Therefore, it can be thought that a small dose of strychnos can play a role in dredging collaterals. However, its application is mainly centered on the word "taking unblocked transmission". For the syndrome of common collateral diseases, strychnos can dredging the channels and collaterals and unblocking qi and blood, while for some diseases caused by the accumulation of toxins, such as carbuncle and cancer, strychnos can also reduce the swelling by virtue of its characteristic of taking unblocked transmission.

悟空行医用巴豆
Croton and Emperor Zhuzi

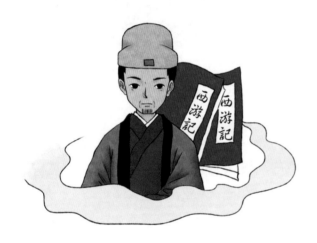

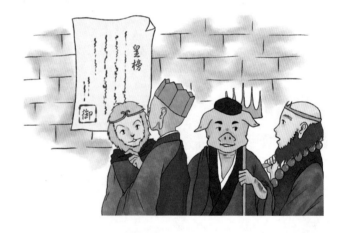

巴豆是自古公认的剧毒之药，而吴承恩的《西游记》却记载有一则孙悟空用巴豆巧治朱紫国国王的故事。

Croton has been believed to be a highly toxic medicine in ancient times. In Wu Cheng'en's *Journey to the West* recorded a story of Wukong skillfully treating Emperor of Zhuzi with croton.

书中记载，唐僧师徒四人途经朱紫国，却发现国王久病难愈，不能上朝，只好贴出皇榜张榜寻医。

When the Tang Priest and his disciples were passing through the kingdom of Zhuzi, they found that the emperor was unable to go to imperial court because of a lingering illness. The court had to post an emperor notice for highly skilled doctors.

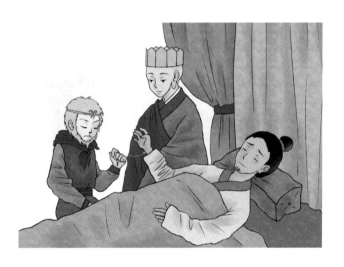

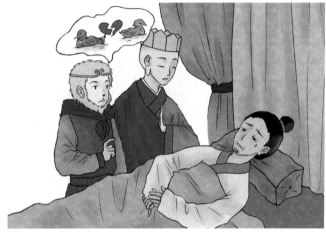

孙悟空曾在菩提祖师门下习得医术，便揭了皇榜，进宫为国王悬丝诊脉。

Since Wukong had once learned medical skills from Master Puti, he took off the imperial notice and entered the palace to feel the emperor's pulse through suspended threads.

悟空诊断国王所患为双鸟失群之症，认为是鸳鸯分飞的相思所致，但当先治其标。

Wukong diagnosed that the emperor's disease was actually a psychological problem and that it was caused by his separation from his wife. However, he believed that the priority was to relieve the patient's symptoms.

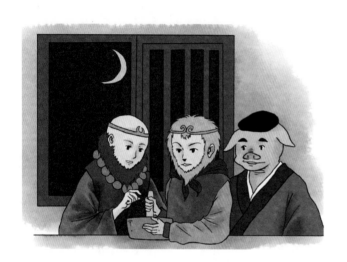

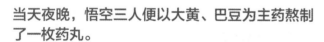

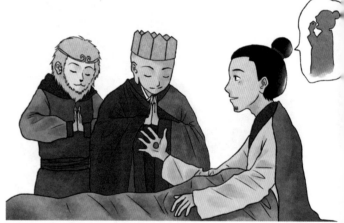

当天夜晚，悟空三人便以大黄、巴豆为主药熬制了一枚药丸。

On that night, Wukong and his two fellows decocted a pill with two main drugs—rhubarb and croton.

第二日，国王服药之后，从大便排出许多秽污痰涎，顿时感觉精神振奋了许多。

The next day, after the emperor took the pill, he pooped a great deal of dirty phlegm and immediately felt refreshed.

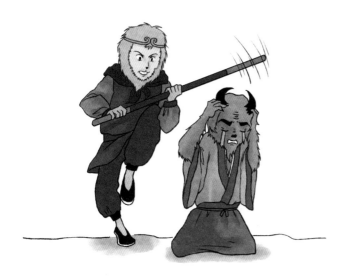

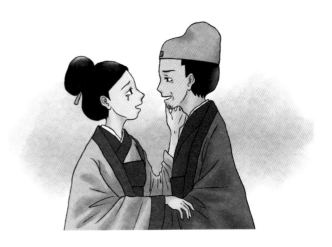

之后，为了解国王的心病，孙悟空打败了妖怪赛太岁，救回了金圣娘娘。

Later, in order to treat the emperor's mental illness, Wukong defeated the Monster Saitaisui and saved Empress Jinsheng, the wife of the emperor.

从此，夫妻团聚，国王的病也彻底痊愈了。

From then on, the couple reunited and the emperor's illness was completely cured.

巴豆功效
The Efficacy of Croton

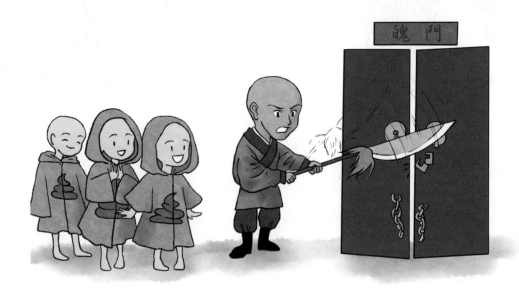

功效分析

巴豆广为人知的是其作为毒药的身份，但它却也是历代医家手中的治病良药。故事中的朱紫国国王患相思之疾，肝郁不疏而气机阻滞，积滞痰涎久居胃肠不得运化，治疗应以涤除久积为先。巴豆被誉为斩关夺门之将，属峻下之药，国王胃肠得通，气机得畅，自然精神也就好了大半。目前认为，巴豆性辛热，可峻下冷积，逐水消肿，主要用于寒积便秘，腹水鼓胀的治疗。

Efficacy Analysis

Croton is widely known as a poison, but it was also used as a good medicine by doctors of past dynasties. In the story, the emperor suffered from lovesickness, causing the stagnation of liver qi which led to the stagnation of qi. And the stagnation of qi further triggered the stagnation of phlegm which could not be transported and dissolved but stayed in the stomach and intestine for a long term. The stagnation should be washed away first. Croton is reputed to be the most powerful medicine in drastic purgatives. After taking it, the emperor felt unobstructed in the stomach and intestine, showing that his qi was unblocked so that his natural spirit was much better. At present, it is believed that croton is pungent and hot and that it can expel cold accumulation, purge water and relieve swelling, so it is mainly used for the treatment of constipation due to cold accumulation and ascites distension.